Gestational Diabetes & You

Text Copyright © 2019 Dr. Mary-S. Echols, RN, BSN,MSN, DNP

For more information on bulk orders, book sponsorships, speaking engagements or workshops, please send all correspondence to :

TAAP,LLC, P.O. Box 47086, Oak Park,MI 48237

Published by:

The Amazing Adventures of Pregnancy (TAAP),LLC

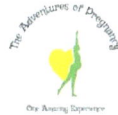

Oak Park, MI

By Dr. Mary Echols,RN, DNP,MSN,BSN
Edited by Tenita Johnson

Library of Congress Control Number
2020908643

Gestational Diabetes & You by Mary Echols -- [1st ed.].

"Gestational Diabetes & You"
Paperback ISBN: 978-1-7350094-0-7
Ebook ISBSN:978-1-7350094-1-4

First Edition
Printed in the U.S.A.

This book is dedicated to all pregnant women, especially those with Gestational Diabetes who have crossed my path-may they realize they are stronger and more Amazing then they realize.

To my parents, Mary Ann & Orzell, who are my biggest cheerleaders in life and truly the wind beneath my wings; thank you for pushing me to soar. To my husband Stephen, for his support and for thinking I can literally move mountains. Last but not least my baby girl, Mary Beth; my world who inspires me to be better every day! I love you to the moon and back!

A Note to Readers

Finally, my desire is you are empowered on your journey with Gestational Diabetes. That you will not fear - but embrace this journey with knowledge and understanding as you form a partnership with your provider to have a healthy pregnancy and a healthy baby.

Please visit the following Facebook page and hit like to join a community of Mothers and Mothers –to –be on their Pregnancy Journey

The Amazing Adventures of Pregnancy
https://www.facebook.com/theamazingadventuresofpregnancy/

Please feel free to send an email to "GDM" in subject line. I will be happy to answer any questions or email you any updated/edition of this book (Ebook only, not printed) completely free as thanks for purchasing this book. I look forward to hearing your suggestions and input.

Introduction

When you learned that you had gestational diabetes, did you feel confused, worried or angry? If you had any of these feelings, it is okay. These are all normal feelings for a new diagnosis.

The good news is that gestational diabetes can be controlled. A commitment from you and a partnership with your healthcare providers can result in a healthy pregnancy and healthy baby.

Your high-risk doctor and OB-GYN will create a plan of care just for you and your needs because each woman and situation are different. This booklet will help guide you in learning how to live with gestational diabetes.

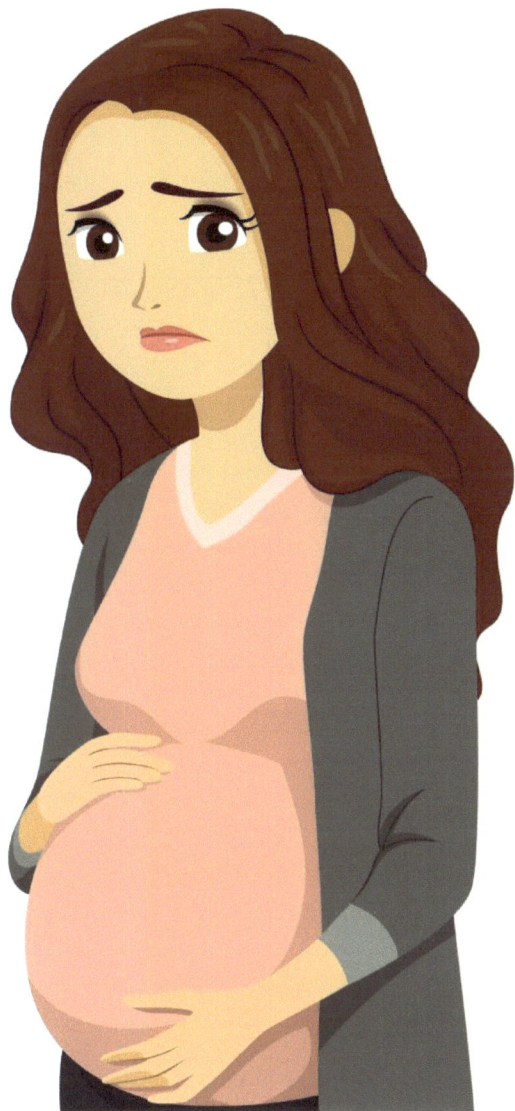

What is Gestational Diabetes?

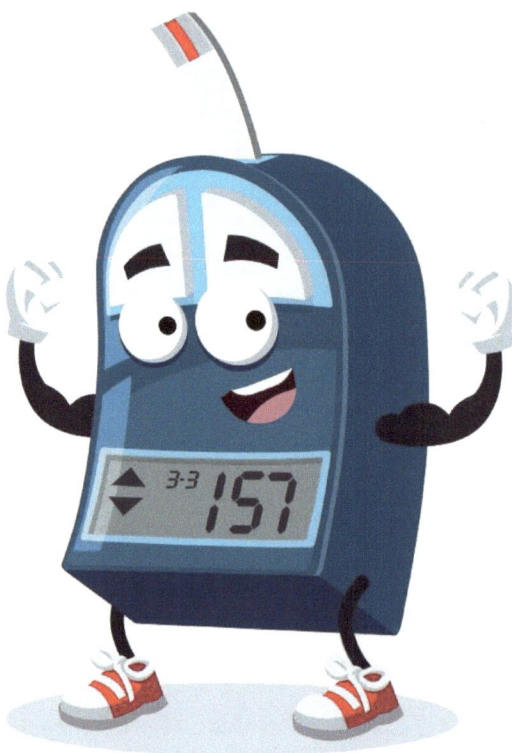

Gestational (jes-tay-shun-ul) diabetes is a type of diabetes that occurs during pregnancy. A woman is usually diagnosed with gestational diabetes between 24-28 weeks of pregnancy. This diagnosis suggests that the body is using too little insulin in the pancreas or cannot make enough insulin (Center for Disease Control [CDC], 2018).

Insulin is a hormone in your body that keeps your blood sugar in control. The lack of insulin causes the blood glucose (blood sugar) to become too high and extra sugar collects in the blood. This glucose (sugar) stays in the blood instead of being used for energy (CDC, 2017). This extra sugar in your blood can be harmful to you and your baby. However, gestational diabetes can be managed through your meal planning. You may also need medication, insulin or pills. Your doctor will help you develop a plan.

It is very important to start treatment quickly when you are diagnosed with gestational diabetes, as it can be harmful to you and your baby (The American Diabetes Association [ADA], 2014).

Are You at Risk for Gestational Diabetes?

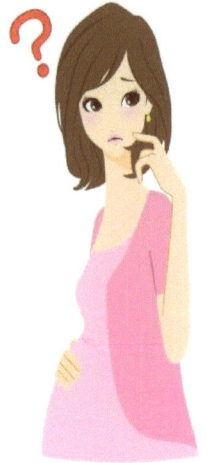

Any female who is pregnant can develop gestational diabetes.
Remember, developing gestational diabetes is not your fault. Every
year, 2-10% of women develop gestational diabetes in the United States
(CDC, 2017).

You are at risk for developing gestational diabetes if:

- You have delivered at least one baby weighing more than nine pounds.

- You are overweight.

- You have a history of gestational diabetes with a previous pregnancy.

- Your family has a history of Type 2 diabetes.

- You are African American/Asian-American, Hispanic/Latin or Pacific Islander.

- You are 25 or older.

    (CDC, 2017)

How Does Gestational Diabetes Affect You?

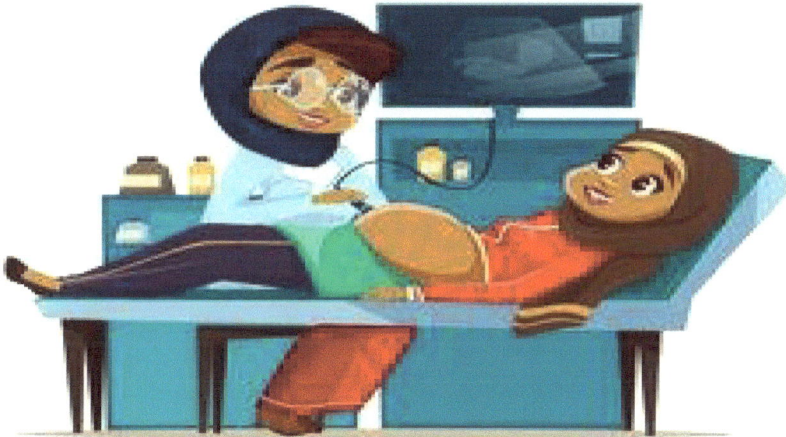

With gestational diabetes, you are considered "high risk," which means you and your baby will be watched very closely by your doctor for the duration of your pregnancy.

With gestational diabetes, you are at risk for:

- Developing Type 2 diabetes in the future
- Developing high blood pressure

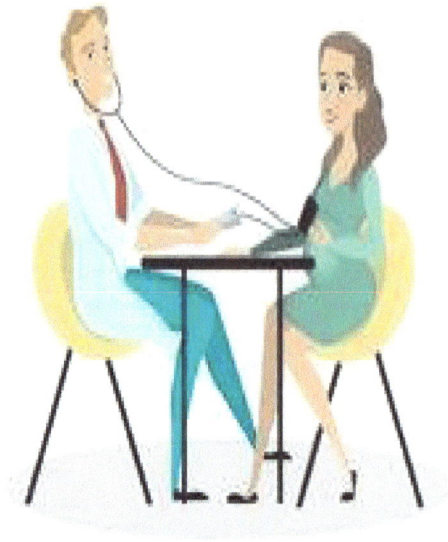

- **Delivering a *big* baby, which means you may need a Cesarean section (C-section), which is a surgical procedure to deliver your baby manually (CDC, 2017).**

Yes, these are scary facts. However, remember that, between you and your doctor, gestational diabetes can be managed. Also, gestational diabetes normally goes away after delivery.

You should be tested for diabetes 6-12 weeks after your baby is born. It is also encouraged that you have consistent visits with your primary doctor to make sure your levels are within normal limits (CDC, 2017).

Will My Baby Be Okay?

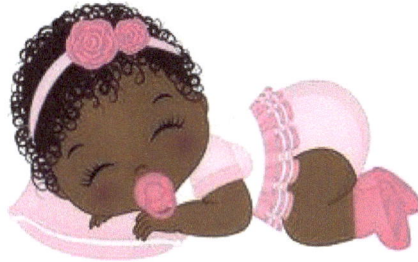

The biggest question you are probably asking yourself is:

Will my baby be okay?

When you have gestational diabetes, your baby's health is at risk for several things:

- Your baby is at risk for weighing more than the average-size newborn, making birth difficult.

- Your baby may be born with a low blood sugar and will need close medical supervision while in the hospital. The baby may also be admitted to the NICU.

- Your baby may have difficulty breathing.

- Your baby may develop Type 2 diabetes in the future.

However, many babies of mothers with gestational diabetes are born healthy. Maintaining blood sugar control during your pregnancy can result in delivering a healthy baby.

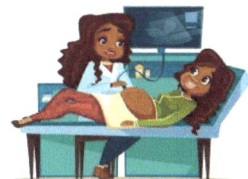

What is the NICU?

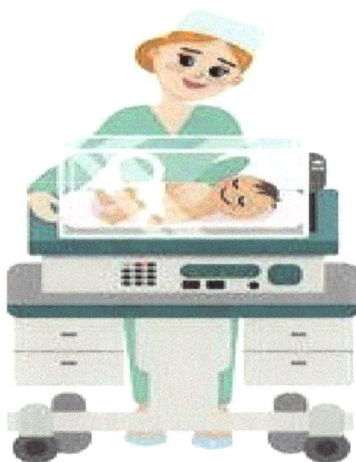

The Neonatal Intensive Care Unit (NICU) is a unit in the hospital, usually near the Labor and Delivery area, where a team is available to provide excellent care for your baby. The babies in the NICU are closely observed by the nurses and doctors 24/7.

A baby born to a mother who has gestational diabetes *may* have breathing problems or low blood sugar. If your baby experiences any trouble after delivery, he/she will go to the NICU.

Your baby will most likely stay in the NICU for 24-48 hours. Sometimes, your baby will only have to stay a few hours in the NICU until they are stable. You are allowed to visit your baby while he/she is in the NICU.

Keep in mind that not every baby has to go to the NICU. Your baby will only need the NICU If he/she is having difficulty transitioning from birth. If he/she is not having difficulty, the baby will stay with you after birth.

Meal Planning

When you have gestational diabetes, it is crucial that you maintain a healthy, balanced diet (CDC, 2017).

Your diet should include a variety of food groups, including fruits and vegetables.

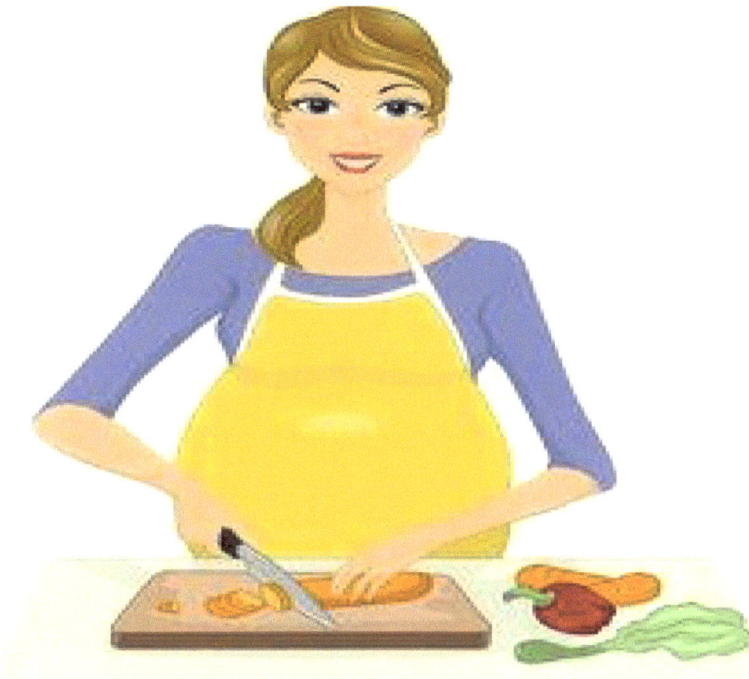

For the health of you and your baby, it is best to avoid, or limit, the amount of regular (sugary) soda, sweets, juices and fast food.

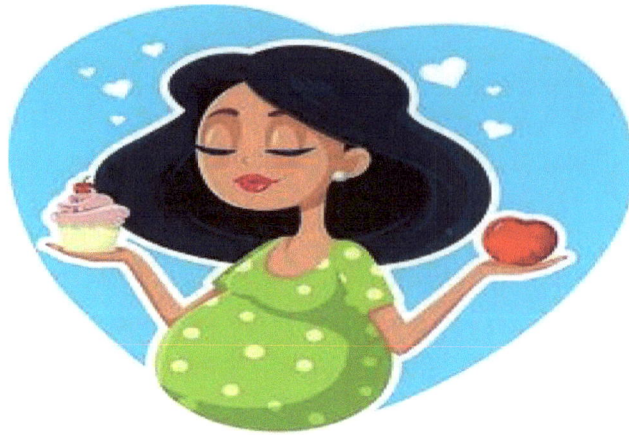

You may have the opportunity to meet with a dietician. This meeting is not meant to put you on a diet, but to help you learn how to manage your food portions, proteins and carbohydrates to yield the best outcome for you and your baby. The dietician can also help you plan your meals to keep your blood sugar levels under control.

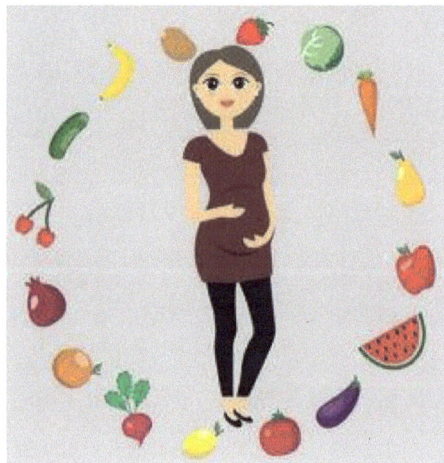

Remember, being a gestational diabetic does not mean you have to starve. It is important that you eat consistently throughout the day. If you do not eat enough, or if your blood glucose results get too high, your body might make *ketones*.

Having ketones in your blood or urine means your body is using fat for energy instead of sugar. This can be harmful to your health, as well as the health of your baby.

Be sure to speak with your healthcare provider regarding your meal plans to make sure you are eating the right foods at the right time (https://www.niddk.nih.gov/health-information/diabetes/overview/what-is-diabetes/gestational/management-treatment).

Staying Active

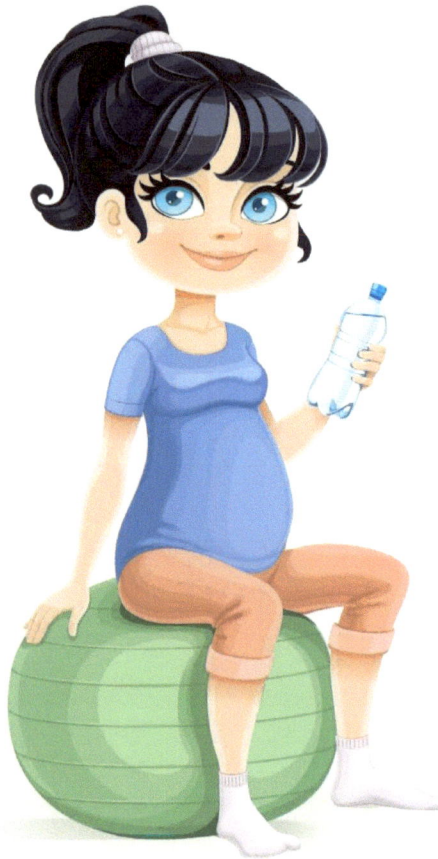

Keep it moving (of course, with your doctor's approval)!

Exercise can be helpful with keeping your blood sugar levels normal.

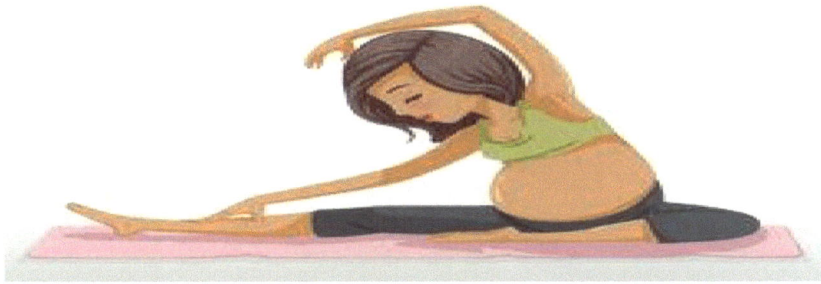

Typically, 30 minutes of moderate-intensity aerobic exercise at least five days a week is recommended. Walking is also a great exercise, especially 10-15 minutes after each meal (The American College of Obstetricians and Gynecologists [ACOG], 2017).

Exercise at least 30 minutes daily. Some other ways you can stay active are:

- Swimming
- Walking
- Stationary
- Bicycling

Remember to speak with your doctor or midwife to determine what is *safe and appropriate* for you and your baby.

Nurse Tips for Taking Care of Yourself

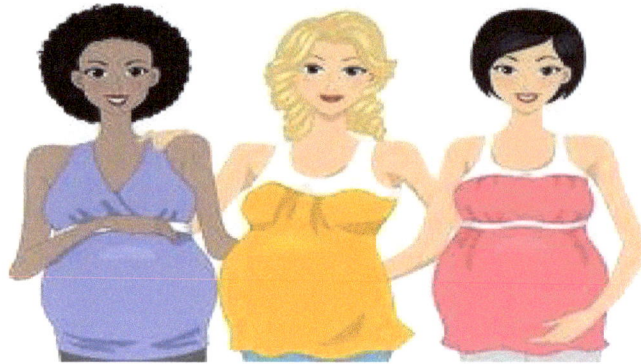

Be kind to yourself!

Do not judge yourself for having gestational diabetes. The main goal is to have a healthy mom and healthy baby. Remember, you have the power to keep you and your baby healthy during your pregnancy.

One way to stay healthy is to keep your blood sugar level under control by:

- **Following your doctor's advice**

- **Seeing your doctor regularly**

- **Checking your blood sugar often**

- **Treating any signs of low blood sugar quickly**

How do you check your glucose results?

Now that you have learned about gestational diabetes, it's important to know what you need to monitor your glucose levels.

The following is a list of supplies you will need to check your glucose levels:

- Glucometer
- Testing Strips
- Lancets
- Lancet Device

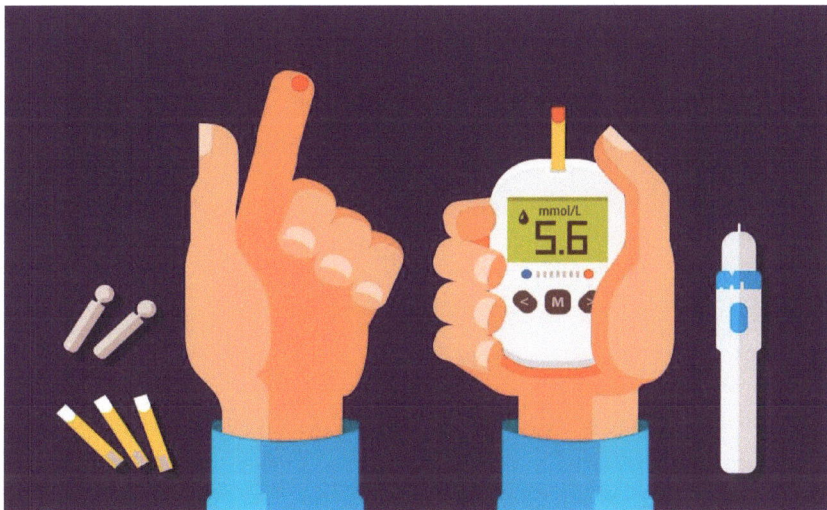

- Alcohol Swabs
- Log Sheet or Book
- *Your Doctor's Guidelines***

Steps to Check Your Glucose Results

1. Clean your finger with an alcohol swab.
2. Insert a new lancet into the lancet device.
3. Insert the test strip.
4. Poke your finger.
5. Place blood onto the test strip.
6. Discard your lancet into the Sharps Container.
7. Read and document.

Tips for Collecting Blood for Test Strips

1. Warm your finger up.
2. Milk your finger from the side.
3. Collect blood from the side of your finger.
4. Use the second drop of blood.

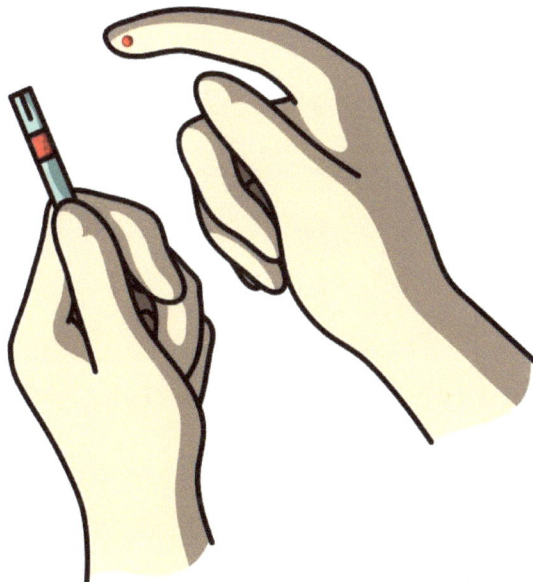

Diabetes Log Sheet

It is important that you monitor your blood sugar often. Speak with your doctor or midwife about how often you will need to monitor your glucose levels, and when you need to have your provider review your results.

You should try to keep your blood sugars at or below:

	The level my doctor recommends	
When Fasting	____mg/dL or lower	
1 or 2 hours after meals	____mg/dL or lower	

*Ask your doctor what he/she would like your glucoses to be, and if you should check one or two hours after meals.

You may have a glucose log sheet from your doctor or one that comes in your diabetes testing supply kit. However, please feel free to use this glucose log sheet I have created. Copy as many as you need.

Glucose Log Sheet

Date	Fasting	2 Hours After Breakfast	2 Hours After Lunch	2 Hours After Dinner	Insulin/ Medication	Snacks

High Blood Sugar

When your blood sugar readings are high, you can experience symptoms of hyperglycemia, which include:

- **Thirst**

- **Blurred vision**

- **Headaches**

- **Frequent urination**

- **Feel weak or tired**

- **Difficulty paying attention**

    (https://www.niddk.nih.gov/health-information/diabetes/overview/managing-diabetes)

Ask your doctor or nurse what you should do if your blood sugar is high.

Write the instructions here for later reference:

Low Blood Sugar

When your blood sugar readings are low, you may feel symptoms of low blood sugar (hypoglycemia) which include, but are not limited to:

- **Dizziness**
- **Sweating**
- **Hunger**
- **Headache**
- **Pale skin color**
- **Sudden moodiness or behavior changes, such as crying for no apparent reason**
- **Clumsy or jerky movement**
- **Seizures**
- **Difficulty paying attention or confusion**
- **Tingling sensations around your mouth**
- **The feeling that your heart is beating too fast**

If you have these symptoms, you must act quickly! Check your blood sugar. If it is below your target of what you and your doctor have discussed, eat or drink 15 grams of carbohydrates right away. Wait 15 minutes and recheck your glucose level.

(https://www.niddk.nih.gov/health-information/diabetes/overview/preventing-problems/low-blood-glucose-hypoglycemia)

It is important to be aware of what to do *before* it happens. Be sure to talk to your provider about what you should do in this situation.

Tips for Treating Low Blood Sugar (Hypoglycemia)

- **When your blood sugar is low, it is *crucial* that you treat yourself quickly.**

- **Check your blood sugar, and eat or drink 15 grams of carbohydrates *immediately*!**

Sources that will treat low blood sugar quickly are:

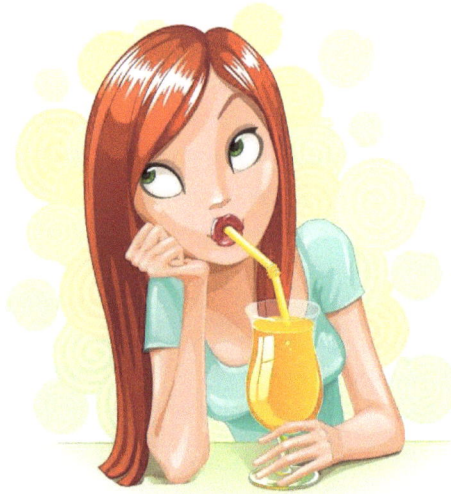

4 oz. (1/2 cup) of juice or regular soda

1 cup of milk

2 tablespoons of raisins

4-5 saltine crackers

4 teaspoons of sugar

1 tablespoon of honey or corn syrup

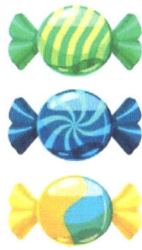

Hard Candies (*crunch*, not suck)

Once you have checked your blood sugar level, and you have treated your low blood sugar with one of the suggestions above, check your blood sugar level again. If your blood sugar level is still low, and your symptoms do not go away, eat a source of sugar again.

*Call your doctor if your blood sugar is lower than _____.

(*Ask your doctor to write in the number*)

After you feel better, be sure to eat regular meals as you and your dietician planned, and keep your glucose within normal range

(https://www.niddk.nih.gov/health-information/diabetes/overview/preventing-problems/low-blood-glucose-hypoglycemia)

Take Control of Your Diagnosis (Checklist)

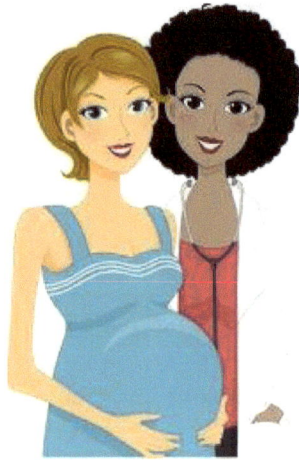

- Educate yourself and be informed of your diagnosis. Ask questions and write down the answers.

- Schedule all of your prenatal doctor and ultrasound appointments in advance. It reduces stress of trying to schedule at the last minute.

- Try to meal plan/prep. It makes sticking to a healthy diet easier.

- Stick to a schedule. Check your blood sugar and eat your meals at the same time daily.

- If you take medication, write down the time and dose you are taking.

- Keep your diabetic testing supplies in a small carrying case so you can keep it with you at all times.

- Know your blood sugar levels. Ask your doctor what the normal levels are for you.

- Know the signs and symptoms of hypoglycemia and hyperglycemia.

- Be kind to yourself.

- Be sure to schedule "me time" and "self-care" time.

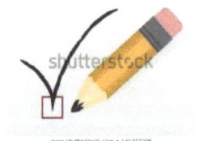

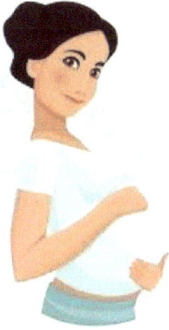

Will I Need Special Tests?

Depending on your diagnosis, your doctor may or may not order all of these tests.

- **Kick Counts:**
    This is a record of how often you feel the fetus move. Your doctor typically has you start this around 32 weeks' gestation. Be sure to ask your doctor how often your baby should move.

- **Non-Stress Test (NSTs):**
    This test measures your baby's heart rate to make sure your baby is not under stress. This test is typically started around 32 weeks' gestation. This test is done in the hospital or your doctor's office. You will be placed in a chair or bed and have belts with a sensor placed around your abdomen. A machine will record the baby's heart rate and determine whether or not you're having contractions.

Biophysical Profile (BPP):
    This test monitors the fetal heart rate using an ultrasound exam. The BPP checks the fetus' heart rate and estimates the amount of amniotic fluid, the baby's breathing, movement and muscle tone.

    (The American College of Obstetricians and Gynecologists [ACOG], 2017)

Healthy Pregnancy/Healthy Baby

       Gestational diabetes is a cause for concern; however, there is good news. You can work together with your healthcare team, including your doctor/obstetrician, nurse, educator and dietician to keep your glucose results within normal levels. This will allow you to manage your gestational diabetes successfully.

       Working together as a team will result in a healthy pregnancy and a healthy baby.

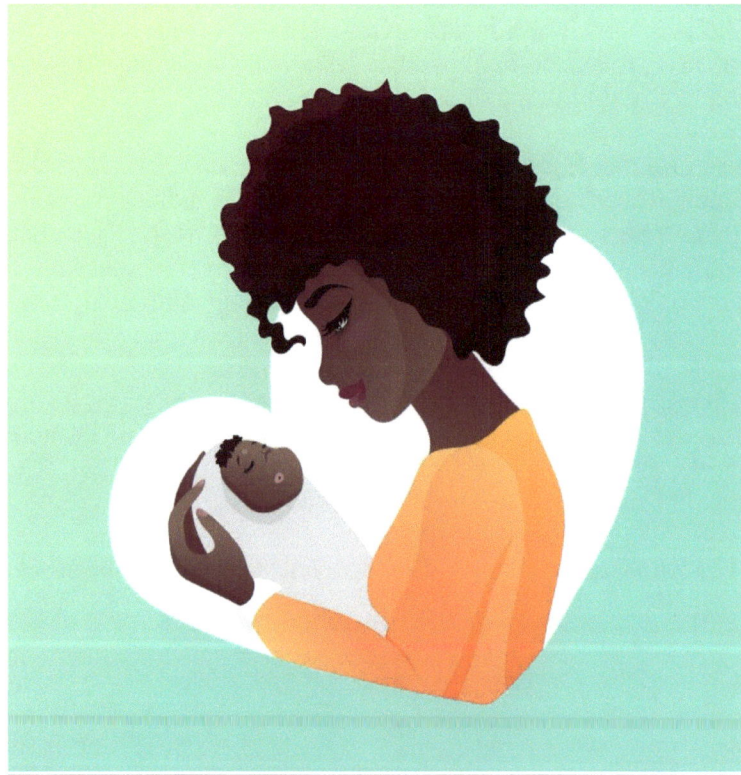

References

American Diabetes Association. (2016). What is Gestational Diabetes. *Retrieved from*
  http://diabetes.org/diabetes-basics/gestational/what-is-gestational-diabetes.html

American Diabetes Association. (2014). How to Treat Gestational Diabetes. *Retrieved from*
  http://www.diabetes.org/diabetes-basics/gestational/how-to-treat-gestational.html

Centers for Disease Control and Prevention. (2017). Gestational Diabetes. *Retrieved from*
  https://www.cdc.gov/diabetes/basics/gestational.html

Centers for Disease Control and Prevention. (2018). Gestational Diabetes and Pregnancy. *Retrieved*
  from https://www.cdc.gov/pregnancy/diabetes-gestational.html

Farahvar, S., Walfisch, A. & Sheiner, E. (2018). Gestational diabetes risk factors and long term
  consequences for both mother and offspring: a literature review. *Expert Review of*
  Endocrinology & Metabolism. DOI: 10.1080/17446651.2018.1476135

National Institute of Diabetes and Digestive and Kidney Diseases ([NIDDK]).(2016).Low Blood
Glucose
  (Hypoglycemia). U.S. Department of Health and Human Services. Retrieved from
  https://www.niddk.nih.gov/health-information/diabetes/overview/preventing-problems/low-
  blood-glucose-hypoglycemia. The National Institute of Diabetes and Digestive Kidney
  Diseases Health Information Center.

National Institute of Diabetes and Digestive and Kidney Diseases (2017). Managing & Treating

  Gestational Diabetes. How can I manage my gestational diabetes? U.S. Department of
  Health and Human Services. *Retrieved from*
  https://www.niddk.nih.gov/health-information/diabetes/overview/what-is-
  diabetes/gestational/management-treatment. The National Institute of Diabetes and
  Digestive Kidney Diseases Health Information Center.

Padayachee, C., Coombes, J.S. (2015). Exercise guidelines for gestational diabetes mellitus. *World*
  *Journal of Diabetes.*6(8): 1033-1044. Doi:10.4239/wjd.v6.i8.1033

The American College of Obstetricians and Gynecologist [ACOG]. (2017).Patient Education.
  Gestational Diabetes. *Retrieved from h*tps://www.acog.org/Patients/FAQs/Gestational-
  Diabetes

www.ingramcontent.com/pod-product-compliance
Lightning Source LLC
Chambersburg PA
CBHW041245040426
42445CB00005B/144